I0436973

VALAWAUGN BLACKMON MCCAIN

FIGHT FOR YOUR LIFE

The Journey

outskirts
press

Fight For Your Life
The Journey
All Rights Reserved.
Copyright © 2017 Valawaugn Blackmon McCain
v3.0

The opinions expressed in this manuscript are solely the opinions of the author and do not represent the opinions or thoughts of the publisher. The author has represented and warranted full ownership and/or legal right to publish all the materials in this book.

This book may not be reproduced, transmitted, or stored in whole or in part by any means, including graphic, electronic, or mechanical without the express written consent of the publisher except in the case of brief quotations embodied in critical articles and reviews.

Outskirts Press, Inc.
http://www.outskirtspress.com

ISBN: 978-1-4787-9073-0

Cover Photo © 2017 thinkstockphotos.com. Author Photo © 2017 Ayinde Simpson. All rights reserved - used with permission.

Outskirts Press and the "OP" logo are trademarks belonging to Outskirts Press, Inc.

PRINTED IN THE UNITED STATES OF AMERICA

ACKNOWLEDGMENTS

To the only wise God my Lord and Savior Jesus Christ, Thank you for allowing me to live twenty-one years! To my mother Betty Jewel Tatum, my children Deontre Juwaugn Newkirk, Nyshia Lashay Bennett, and Isaiah Nysheed Bennett, thank you for all of the love and support through the years. This book is dedicated to you, my family, and all the others that have helped me along the way. To the doctors that have taken care of me for twenty-one years, thank you! To Apostle Carolyn L. Hicks (Deliverance Jesus Is Coming Victory Center) for allowing God to use you! First Baptist Church for having a benefit service to aid in my recovery, & ST. Thomas A.M.E. Zion Church Roseboro NC. my home church for your prayers. To all of my family and friends that helped me along the way, thank you!

INTRODUCTION

This is not going to be your ordinary book! I am not a scholar, nor am I a world renowned author. I am Valawaugn a woman who grew up in a small community outside of Roseboro NC called Highsmith Side. I grew up walking the dirt roads as most children did back then. My childhood was not like most but that's another story for another time. We will fast forward to why I am writing this book in the first place.

The purpose of this book is to give people hope! To let people of all walks of life, all colors, creeds, cultures, and nationalities, know that you do not have to die from cancer, lupus, or any other disease. This may sound funny to you as you may be saying to yourself, people do die in fact some of my family members have died! This may be true and I am not arguing that fact. Yes, some die because God has a bigger and better job for them to do but most, hear me out, GIVE UP. Many people lose the will to live! They think about the road ahead and it is very uncertain. Many have no faith to run to, a God to pray to, so they give up. Many do not want to go through treatments or be under the doctor's care. I write this book for all of you! I write this book for all of the survivor's! To the supporters and doctors you are my heroes! This book is to get you off your seat of do nothing and live! That diagnoses is not the end, it is just the beginning of a new, better, and different life! I am not saying it is going to be easy but IT IS DOABLE! I write this book from my thoughts, what I have learned and may paraphrase scriptures out of the bible throughout this book. I am not trying to accredit it to myself but only try to live what I have read and I speak it over my life. I believe my faith in God has gotten me where I am today and this book prophesized so long ago that I would write, is now in your hands. Come take this Journey with me!

TABLE OF CONTENTS

Chapter 1

~~~

THE BEGINNING

I WAS A senior at Lakewood High School I was nineteen years old and pregnant! Yep that's right, I was forty four weeks over due! I know, I know you may be thinking all sorts of things but, the fact of the matter is that I wasn't the first girl to be pregnant at a young age and I sure won't be the last. I was faithful at taking the pill and using protection this was just what happened. I don't make excuses for myself and I would tell any young girl to save themselves for marriage. Taking care of a baby is not easy as your whole life changes. Again that is another story for another time.

The time came for me to be induced because my blood pressure began to rise and I was too many weeks overdue. I was admitted into the hospital at 6am on October 24, 1995 and was put on what many call the drip. The drip is the medications used to make you have contractions and dilate. At first it didn't hurt too badly, it was like a menstrual cramp and the little Braxton Hicks contractions, I was having prior to going into labor. As the hours past the contractions seem to be more than I could bear. The doctor came around periodically and checked me, but after several hours I had not dilated but two centimeters. As I laid there in the worst pain on this side of heaven my doctor from my knowledge went home to take a nap because he did not see me having my baby any time soon. I remember being in so much pain that all I could do was clutch my stomach and cry. As more hours passed my blood pressure began to rise, both numbers were in the three digits and my head began to hurt. The machines I was on started to beep and my head now started to burn! It felt like someone had set fire to it and I was in so much pain, that I was numb! I remember hearing the nurses saying call the doctor and my mom asking what was going on; then all of a sudden I heard nothing, all of my pain was gone, I was at peace. It felt like I was in another place. I remember closing my eyes as the nurse started the third IV.

In that instance I knew I was dying. I told my mother to go back to certain individuals and tell them that I was sorry and to ask for them to forgive me! I told her that it was ok I didn't feel pain anymore. I told her that I was ok but then something happened! My mom placed her hand on my head and immediately I was in excruciating pain again and my head was about to explode. They told me that my baby was in stress and had made a bowel movement inside of me. The nurse began to suction around my son. She told me that I needed to hold on. I know that it was the hand of God on me as I drifted several times. As my mom would lift her hand, I would drift as she placed her hand back on my head, I would comeback. I remember hearing in the mist of all of the pain her saying, "If my baby dies all of you will be sued!" The nurse went under the covers to check me and again called for the doctor; but he was nowhere to be found and they called a surgeon in for me.

The surgeon had not yet arrived, and because my baby had a bowel movement in me he was in stress. The nurses were very concerned for his safety. All of a sudden they started getting these suction tubes and suctioning the feces from around my baby and telling me to keep calm. I began to tell them again, that my head was burning and they assured me that it was the blood pressure medications that was the cause of it.

Finally, the doctor arrives and checks me and immediately says there is no way she can have this baby! Prep her for surgery!

He comes to the side of my bed and says you're going to be ok! He told me that he had to give me a cesarean section better known as a C-Section. I was in so much pain I just wanted it to be over! I was terrified! They prepped me and rushed me to the operating room and then the doctor drops the bomb on me! He tells me that I cannot be put to sleep because of my blood pressure, that I could go to sleep and never wake up! What! Wait a minute I have to be awake? He then began to explain that he was going to give me a spinal tap in my back to numb my body from the waist down. He said that I had to lay on my side real still and be careful not to move. I remember thinking to myself, don't move! I am in so much pain all I can do is rock from side to side! There were two nurses in front of me one held my shoulders and the other my legs. The doctor of course, was behind me. I was so scared I just wanted it all to be over. As I was laying on my side the doctor said hold real still you're going to feel several little pinches. Again I thought to myself, I am already in so much pain just do it! Why did I say that he stuck me in my back and it felt like someone was poking me with three needles all at the same time in my spine.

The nurses rolled me over and instantly I felt no more pain. The doctors kept asking could I feel anything and my answer was no. They also kept saying that it was going to be just a little bit longer. Finally I heard a cry and the doctor said You Have A Baby Boy! I had my son at 11:42pm on October 24, 1995 he was 8 pounds 2&3/4 ounces, and 21 inches long. All I could do was cry as the nurse brought him around to me and placed him up against my cheek. He was all wrinkled and red from his ordeal so they took him and checked him out. The doctor was stitching me up and telling me that I would see my baby soon. He wanted me to get some rest because my blood pressure needed to go down so I did. They took me to my room my mom was there and turned all the lights off and I slept.

The next day they came in and checked me pressed on my stomach and I yelled of course because I had never been cut! They told me that because of my blood pressure, I could not have any visitors and I had to sit in a pitch black room. They did not want me to get excited. Family members came and were turned around at the door only my sons father and my mother could see me. They came to my room and I was finally allowed to get up. The nurse began to help me out of bed and boy was I hurting! It felt like someone struck a match to the bottom of my stomach it burned so bad and stung. The nurse said you have to get up and walk. My motivation was that she was making me walk to go see my son.

As I walked in the baby's area, she directed me to my son. As soon as I saw him I began to cry because he was concealed in this glass case, I could not hold him. There was an opening in the glass where I could put my hands to feel his hands. He had small red blisters on his face and body. The nurse told me he was sick from the feces that was on him and that they had to monitor him and suction his mouth when he was born. She assured me I would hold him soon they just had to check him out completely first.

Day three they allowed my son to come to my room. This was the happiest day of my life. He was so small and his eyes were so big! He looked just like his dad. The following day we both were released from the hospital. I was happy to be finally going home to recover and enjoy my new buddle of Joy! So I thought!

Chapter 2

LATE IN THE MIDNIGHT HOUR

I ARRIVED HOME and was very sore my mother told me to lay down and she would take care of my son. Oh by the way I named him Deont're Juwaugn Newkirk. Two days had past and I still was sore but I could move around a little better. My son's father had come down to see him and myself because of course I couldn't go out. My mom was a stickler for that staying in the house six weeks deal and it was cold outside too; I didn't have a chance. My son's father watched him because I had only been home for two days and was still very weak; I was tired so I went to lay down. I slept on into the night. I remember tossing and turning in my sleep because my head was hurting. I woke up and called for my mom who was on the other end of the house caring for my son. I began to regurgitate.

My mom ran back to the room where I was and saw that I was re-gurgitating bile. From her experience at the hospital as a nurse aide she knew there was something terribly wrong. I had the worst headache of my life! It hurt all over! The lights were too bright and I had to keep a trash bag near. She helped me get dressed and we with my son, went back to the hospital. At the hospital they took me in the back, and made me change into a gown so that they could check me because I had just given birth not even a week prior. I was trying to tell them my head was the problem but every time I opened my mouth I threw up! The doctor ordered blood test to see if I had infection somewhere and also ordered a head CAT scan.

I was taken to get the CAT scan, and to move from one table to another felt like someone was clawing at my stomach all I could do was cry! The person taking the scan apologized because she knew I was in pain because of the incision under my stomach and to bend back and forth was painful. Now because of this ordeal my head as well as my stomach was hurting. I was now hurting all over. They returned me back to my room and gave me something for pain, needless to say it didn't work. All I could do was look at my son with tears in my eyes. He was nestled in his car seat asleep. My mom placed the seat at the foot of my bed and sat on the corner beside me. I saw the worry in her eyes as she would rub my head. I remember as a little girl when I would have asthma attacks she would rub my head to calm me down and now to this day it still works! She looked at me and said it will be alright they will find out what is wrong. I knew by the way she said it that she was hoping I would be ok because she almost lost me in child birth.

The doctor comes in the room with a look on his face that told me right then that something was wrong! He called my mom out of the room and I began to get hysterical and told them to come back in because I wanted to hear what was wrong with me! My mom walked back in the room and the doctor plus two nurses walked in behind him. He told me that the nurses was going to start IV's on me. They proceeded to stick me on already sore arms three times. The doctor said that I had abnormalities on my brain. I looked at him and then at my mom as she was trying to be strong. The doctor looked at my mom and asked her where did she want me to be sent? Sent? I said. He said yes, then began to say the name of two hospitals but to keep those hospitals confidential we will just say hospital C & D? My mom replied, C. After about three hours an ambulance from C arrived to take me. Still in pain I was moved once again from one bed to another for transport. Every time I moved I was in pain the burning around my incision was unbearable!

My mom and my son followed the ambulance to hospital C as I was transported; I could feel every bump in the ambulance. Pains shot through my stomach with every turn. Back then they were fixing the roads and they were too much for me. I remember worrying about my son. I was so scared and did not know what was going on. All I could do was cry!

Chapter 3

—✤—

My Arrival

I ARRIVED AT the hospital. The nurses met me and my room was already available in the women's hospital on the maternity floor. The nurse said that in that room I had more privacy because they were told that I had just had my son and he was only six days old. My mom was right behind me as they took me to my room. When I got to it, it was a very large room with a chair bed for my mom and a hospital basinet for my son as well. They brought me a breast pump because I had chosen to breast feed. I remember looking at my baby as tears ran down my face. They left us alone as I fed my son. I remember holding on to him for dear life praying that everything would be alright! My mom came over and sat on the bed and began to rub my head as she always does to calm me down. I saw my baby's big brown eyes as he ate. The nurse came back in while he was eating and said that a doctor had ordered an MRI scan and as soon as my son was finished they would take me.

A guy came in with a wheel chair and said he was taking me to get my test. I was clueless as to what an MRI was so I asked him on the way. He explained to me that it was a tube that you were put in and that you had to lay still for it to take pictures of my brain. I told him that I had a CAT scan and he said yes sort of like that, but that this would be better to see with as it could light up my brain to show the abnormality. When I got to the room there were some ladies there that helped me on this long table that had a sheet draped over it. They rested my head in something that looked like a half of a football helmet with no top. The lady put ear plugs in my ear and told me that I would hear a loud knocking sound and feel the machine shake. I was so scared! She asked if I was claustrophobic and I said no not that I knew of. The lady gave me a ball and said if you need anything squeeze this ball and we will stop the test, but you need to keep real still. She told me that I would be in the MRI for an hour and that I would have dye called contrast going in my IV. I said ok as tears streamed down my face. I remember her wiping my tears and saying we are going to take good care of you.

She pushed a button that slid the table in the MRI. It stopped and there was a light in my eyes. The lady told me to close my eyes because the light could be bright. She then pushed the button again the bed moved. I was in this tube it was so close in there I immediately closed my eyes again and began to say the 23rd Psalm that my mom taught me as a little girl. "The Lord is my shepherd I shall not want he maketh me to lie down into green pastures he leadeth me beside the still waters he restoreith my soul. He leads me in the path for righteousness sake, yea though I walk through the valley of the shadow of death I will fear no evil for tho art with me thy rod and thy staff they comfort me. Tho prepares a table before me in the presence of my enemies my cup runneth over surely goodness and mercy shall follow me all the days of my life and I will dwell in the house of the Lord forever." (The Holy Bible New King James Version, 1994) I kept reciting the scripture over and over. I heard this loud knocking and shaking. I closed my eyes tighter. I kept reciting then all of a sudden I heard a voice inside the MRI that said, we are almost finished but we will now give you the contrast. I said ok. I felt a cold liquid going through my IV. Then all of a sudden I got really warm it felt like I was going to pee on myself. Then I started tasting it, it tasted like I had put a penny in my mouth. I continued to say the 23rd Psalm with tears streaming down my face. Finally the lady comes and says ok you're all done. They pushed me back to my room.

When I got back to the room my mom and son were asleep. I was helped into the bed and I was glad that at least I was with my son and mom. I was told that there would be someone to come and take my blood, but for me to get some rest. I told the nurse that I was hurting and she said that she would ask if I could have pain meds for my head and my stomach incision. I just laid there in that bed starring up at the wall. I did not remember falling asleep. I was awaken when the nurse cut on a bright light over my bed. There was a lady standing over me, she said she had to stick me to draw blood. I was terrified of needles but by this time I just wanted to go back to sleep. They drew about ten tubes of blood. The lady asked me what was my name "Valawaugn Blackmon" I said. She asked what was my date of birth I said, "12/10/76", she looked at the labels that she had, and said thank you then turned the light off and left the room and I went back to sleep.

Chapter 4

━━━━━◆━━━━━

FIFTY/ FIFTY CHANCE

I HEARD A knock at the door. I had no idea how long I was asleep or what time it was when the doctor walked in. He came in with three other people he called them interns. He introduced himself, and allowed the interns to introduce themselves. My mom was holding my son. As he begin to talk, he explained that there was a tumor on my brain. He said that in order to see what kind of tumor it was, I would need to have a brain biopsy. I looked at my mom then back at him. The doctor went on to explain the procedure, he said that he would shave my head right over where the tumor was. I thought to myself SHAVE MY HEAD! Now just to let you know I loved my hair and to shave it was not good. Cut it ok I can deal with that but shave it, I just shook my head. He went on to say that he would have to go inside my brain and get a piece of the tumor and test it. He said that was the only way they could tell if it was malignant or benign. I asked him what those words meant. He told me that it was to see if I had brain cancer or not, that if it was benign that it would not be anything to worry about. I immediately was afraid! I asked my mom for my son and all I could do was hold him in my arms and cry. The doctor told me that if my mom agreed for me to have this done, I would have a fifty/ fifty chance of surviving the biopsy.

Yelp! You heard me right a fifty/ fifty chance! Ok I thought to myself I could die! I asked the doctor if anyone survived the biopsy before and he smiled at me and said yes. He told me and my mom that the brain was complex and sometimes things happen and he wanted to give us all the facts before we agreed or should I say, my mom agree for me to go through it. He said that I could lose my left extremities. Lose what I asked? He said your ability to walk. I was devastated! My doctor assured me that he would do his best to make sure I came through ok. He left the room, so my mom and I could talk about it. My mom asked me what I wanted to do as it was my life. Being a nineteen year old with a new born baby I didn't want to die! She asked me what I wanted and I said to do it. The doctor came in and I asked him; if I didn't get the biopsy what would happen. I remember him telling me that I could possibly die if it was cancer. I thought to myself, If I do this I have a fifty/fifty chance of living if I don't I could just one day die. I told him that we would do the biopsy. He said ok and said that it would be the very next morning. He told us that the faster he could get to it the more answers we would have, and would know what type of tumor it was.

When he left out of the room all I could do was cry! I looked at my son and all I could say was Lord please help me! I held on to him for dear life. All I could do was kiss his cheeks as tears streamed down my face. My mom took him from me and all I could do was lay back in the bed in a fetal position and ball up like a baby. My head begin to hurt, so my mom called the nurse and she brought me some pain medicine. I thought to myself; I could die and leave my baby all alone. My mom came where I was and of course you got it, rubbed my head and said, "it will be alright" I heard the doubt in her voice but to know her and my son was there was comforting.

FIGHT FOR YOUR LIFE

Hours had passed and the nurse came in and told me that the doctor had set the biopsy up for the next morning and I had to be prepped for the surgery. She told me that they would shave my head in the spot the tumor was located. I had very thick long course black hair that went to my shoulders. She placed a towel around my neck and shoulders and picked up some scissors. She began to cut my hair all the way to my scalp. She asked me if I wanted the hair and I told her yes. She then placed it in a small Ziploc bag and handed it to me. She explained that the doctor would finish shaving my head before surgery and clean the area that was to be cut. After she was finished fear set in and all I could do was pray and hold my son. I prayed to God that he would not allow me to die while they did the biopsy. I pleaded that I would see my son and my mom again. I can remember thinking I am too young to be going through this. GOD PLEASE HELP ME!

Chapter 5

——∾∾——

THE INTERN FROM HELL

I RECEIVED A knock on my room door it was the doctor and his team of interns. He asked me was I ready and I remember telling him no. He smiled and said for me not to worry he would do his very best to make sure nothing went wrong. He said he was coming by to make sure I was ok before surgery and he would see me soon. He left the room and immediately fear of dying set in. I grabbed my son and squeezed him real tight without hurting him and kissed him all over his little face. I remember him looking up at me with his big brown eyes. I smiled as my mom took him from me and hugged me. The surgery team knocked on the door with a bed and I got on that bed my mom and son behind me. They took me to an area with curtains and placed me behind it. One of the interns came and said that he had to finish prepping me for my biopsy. The intern had a rolling table with four long needles on it. Ok by this time I AM FREAKING OUT! He told me that the needles contained lidocaine, something that would numb my head for the doctor to do the procedure. I am shaking all over and crying! I absolutely hate needles! He placed his hand on my head and told me to be really still. I griped the arm rail of the bed with both of my hands and bared down on my teeth. The needle felt like a knife going to the base of my skull the medicine burned as it went in! He did two in the front of my head and only one in the back. He brought out a metal contraption that looked like a bird cage by this time I am scared out of my mind. I thought my head is numb so I won't feel anything right? WRONG, he put the bird cage over my head and began to put these long screws in my head as he screwed I felt a lot of pressure. He got two screws in, as he began to put the third screw in on the left side in the back I began to scream telling him it was not numb! I was yelling and hollering telling him my head was burning! He told me it would soon be over just be still. I was waving my hands telling him to get my doctor! I was hysterical! Meanwhile, the doctor could hear me in the operating room and I could see him coming from the back through the double doors. He came over and asked me what was wrong, I told him that he did not numb me all the way because I could feel the screw going in. He pulled the intern away to talk to him. I saw him motion with is hands to leave and seemed very angry. He then came over to me and told the nurse to give me a sedative to calm me down. He gave me the lidocaine and finished putting the screws in my head and securing the halo. He told me that during the surgery I would be awake but in a sleepy state. I said ok and we went into the operating room. They had me to get off the bed and sit in what looked like a small recliner of sorts' black, with a latch on it. I sat down, my head was so heavy because of the halo. He had me to lay back in the recliner and a nurse latched the halo to the chair. As I began to look around all I could see was televisions one in every corner of the room and one right in front of me. I immediately closed my eyes! My doctor placed some head phones on my ears and as I listened I felt myself going to sleep I was hearing classical music. I knew the type of music because I was in the band. It was ok but I was still scared. I heard a sound that I could not make out until.........

Chapter 6

―――∽∾∾―――

It's Burning

IT'S BURNING, IT'S BURNING, I tried to tell the doctor in my sleepy state as he began to drill in my head. Can they hear me I thought, am I asleep? The nurse asked me what's wrong as I could hear the drill and feel it as he cut into my skull! IT'S NOT NUMB I YELLED I'M BURNING. The surgeon immediately stopped and said ok we will numb you some more. Tears were rolling down my cheeks as my head felt like it was on fire. The nurse said calm down we will take care of you, but you have got to calm down. I remember praying to God that he would not let me die. I remember singing, Down at the cross where my Savior died, Down where for cleansing from sin I cried, There to my sin was the blood applied; Glory to His name! Glory to His name, Glory to His name; There to my sin was the blood applied; Glory to His name! (Elisha Albright Hoffman (1839-1929). The more I heard the drill the louder I sung! I remember singing at the cross! At the cross, at the cross where I first saw the light, and the burden of my heart rolled away, it was there by faith I received my sight, and now I am happy all the day!(Ralph Erskine Hudson) (1843-1901). In the mist of me singing the nurse comes and ask am I ok and takes the head phone down from one of my ears. I reply yes but "I feel strange", I told her. She asked me my name I said " Valawaugn Blackmon" She asked me to say my alphabet and I said "A-B-C-D-E-F-G-H-I-J-K-L-M-N-O-P-Q-R-S-T-U-V-W-X-Y-Z" She asked if I could say them backwards and I remember telling her, "I have never been able to do that". The Doctor and the nurse laughed. She placed the head phones back on my ear. I could feel the doctor in my brain picking out the tumor. It felt like, how you pick at a splinter that is embedded in your skin. I began to count every time I felt it but I somehow dozed off and lost count. The nurse came and asked lifting my head phone what is your birthday? I said December 10th 1976. The Doctor said we are almost finished you're doing great! I could feel him stitching me back up because my head would get this tingling sensation. He said all finished and released my head from the seat. It was so heavy. He told me to be real still, that he was going to take what I call the bird cage halo, off. The other nurses that were in the room was holding my arms and two was above my head. They began to unscrew the screws that were in the base of my skull. All of a sudden I got the worst head rush and my brain felt like it was going to explode! I began to yell, scream, and cry! The doctor said we are giving you something for pain it's just your blood going back to where it needs to be. You will be fine your biopsy was a success; now go to your room and rest. I will see you in the morning after your results come back. They pushed me back to my room and my mom greeted me at the door. My head was so heavy but I manage to lift it up just enough to see my son. I reached for him knowing I couldn't hold him. My mom put his face to mine and I motioned for her to put him on the bed with me between my legs as I rubbed his small feet. The nurse came in and said I really needed to rest. My mom came and sat on the bed and rubbed my leg. Her hands always seemed as if it was God himself giving me peace in that storm.

Chapter 7

—❧—

TICK TOCK

I FELT LIKE I had slept for days and my body was so weak. I heard a knock on the hospital door and the doctor walks in with about five interns. He had the strangest look on his face. He stood at the foot of my bed and I knew it was bad news. He looked me straight in my eyes glancing at my mother periodically and said you have a malignant brain tumor. I became numb and thought to myself cancer in my brain! He said it's called an Astrocytoma. It's a stage three inoperable brain tumor which means I can't take it out because of where it was positioned in between your frontal lobes, it's embedded. He went on to explain that this type tumor only goes to stage four before you die. He said they caught it just in time. I began to cry, all I could think about was my son. He asked to speak to my mom out in the hallway and after several minutes of being out there I began to get hysterical! I wanted to know what they were talking about so long. The doctor came in and I asked him and my mom what they were talking about. My mom nodded her head to him for him to tell me. He looked at me and said, "You only have three to five years to live" he went on to say that this tumor was an aggressive tumor and grows very rapidly. He began to tell what my options were to prolong my life, like radiation and chemotherapy but he could not be certain that it would work. He said because I was so young I had a fighting chance than what older adults would have. He was confident in doing both but still was uncertain of the outcome. To find out what happened next, stay on the lookout for the next book Fight For Your Life: The Process as my journey continues!

The Prayer I prayed the night I found out I was dying!

Father God Lord Jesus you made me in my mother's stomach you knew what I would be. You could of taken me on the labor table when I was having my son, why tell me now that I am dying. Why keep me here to hear these words. God what have I done so wrong to deserve a death sentence. I have read your word since I was five years old. God you know what type of home I have grew up in. I have traveled from church to church singing to your glory and also got saved when I was sixteen. God are you punishing me for having sex? God I am no different than most of my friends that have more than one child at my age. God pregnant, I still sung for you and as I laid on that bed for 19 hours I knew I was going to see you why not take me then. I would of never seen his little face. God why now allow me to see him just to take me away from him. God please allow me to see him grow. Allow me to take care of him I'm his mother. Why are you doing this to me what have I done God I don't want to die? I'm only 19, a senior at Lakewood, I don't want to die and leave my baby all alone! Please God hear my prayer and help me! I know your real, I believe you're real! You said if I confess with my mouth the Lord Jesus, and believe in my heart that you raised him from the dead you said, I would be saved. I believe I am saved and your child God. You told me in your bible that if I ask anything in your name I will receive it! So God I'm asking you to heal me so I can take care of my son! Please God In Jesus Name Amen!

Throughout the years I have ran to the bible for many of the answers to the questions I have daily! As a 19 year old I could not go to anyone in my family that had cancer because no one did. While many may not be religious, as for me, I was born and raised in Saint Thomas A.M.E. Zion church where most of the church was family. I traveled in community Choirs and sung songs about God so I knew I could pray to him! I began to go to the New King James version of the bible and find scriptures on healing like Isaiah 53:5 that states "But He was wounded for our transgressions, He was bruised for our iniquities; The chastisement for our peace was upon Him, And by His stripes we are healed." (The Holy Bible New King James Version, 1994) This is the scripture that I live by that I read over and over again. I reminded God in my prayer time with him that He said I was healed. I encourage all of you to do as I did; pray to God for healing remind him of what his word says. Some of you may say that this is not real but it was real for me at 19. It was what I asked God every day when I said my prayers and looked into my sons eyes. This is not the only scripture I read, there were so many more but this one I believe was the mandate given by God concerning my life. I knew he said it I wanted him at 19 to honor it!

Anger set in and the question WHY ME surfaced! I asked God and family members, no one gave me an answer to my question. Despair set in. I was desperate to live but knew in less than five years I would die! Where was this God I grew up loving, praying and singing to? He was nowhere to be found! Does He even hear me? Does he even love me? Does He even care? Family prayed, community prayed, everyone was praying for me!

REFLECTION

I want you now to reflect on your life, on what you may be going through take this page to write it all down.

_____

_____

_____

_____

_____

_____

_____

_____

_____

_____

_____

_____

_____

_____

_____

_____

_____

_____

_____

_____

How do you feel about what you are going through? Be honest with yourself!

_____

_____

_____

_____

_____

_____

_____

_____

_____

_____

_____

_____

_____

_____

_____

_____

_____

_____

_____

_____

_____

_____

_____

_____

_____

_____

What Steps are you going to take to move forward and feel better about the situation? For example, I refused to believe that three to five years was my demise! I got up every day and fought for my life! I dressed myself washed my son and lived, knowing the doctor said I was dying! Write it down and stick to it! THIS IS NOT YOUR END THIS IS YOUR BEGAINING!

_____

_____

_____

_____

_____

_____

_____

_____

_____

_____

_____

_____

_____

_____

_____

_____

_____

_____

_____

_____

_____

_____

_____

Today I feel like.......

_____
_____
_____
_____
_____
_____
_____
_____
_____
_____
_____
_____
_____
_____
_____
_____
_____
_____
_____
_____
_____
_____
_____
_____
_____
_____
_____
_____
_____

Jesus please help me.....

_____

_____

_____

_____

_____

_____

_____

_____

_____

_____

_____

_____

_____

_____

_____

_____

_____

_____

_____

_____

_____

_____

_____

_____

_____

_____

_____

A Prayer

God you are God and my very thoughts you know. You know my pains and my struggles. God you know all things and live in all things including me. Forgive me of my sins. You said by your stipes I am healed and I know through your word I am set free. Cleanse my thoughts and my heart from things that are not like you and forgive me of my sins. I am nothing without you and can do nothing without you holding my hand. Heal me ok from this sickness wash me clean from this infirmity as I know only you can. You are the only one who knows my ending and the length of my days, let them be long and full of joy. If this sickness is unto death help me to learn it and cope always looking to you for strength but it is my desire to be healed from it in Jesus Name. I pull down every stronghold every power, every spiritual wickedness in high places, I cast it down and send it back to the pits of hell from which it came! I decree healing and wholeness, restoration and good health! Show me the way to pray concerning my life, my health and my family keep me in your care under your blood in Jesus Name I pray Amen!

Looking at yourself as God sees you!

Often times we see ourselves as being worthless because of our sicknesses. I am here to tell you that I have been where you are. Sickness is one of those storms that leaves you helpless and hopeless. I need for you to start today saying I am worthy, I am important, I am still of value. I am a soldier, I will learn my sickness and I will conquer this, it will not defeat me. God sees you as more than a conquer he sees you as his child and his friend. As our father he desires to heal you but if he don't then he will give you the strength to stand and fight! I am a living witness to the strength God provides put your trust and faith in him and let him give you peace! It's not over until God says it's over! Not the doctors the almighty God through His son Jesus Christ!

Affirmation's Over My Life

(Say this over your life daily)

I shall live and not die!
Nothing will happen to me today that God doesn't allow!
No matter how I feel I will trust God in this process.
No matter how I feel, I speak healing over my life I will trust God
in this process.
No matter how I feel, I will speak deliverance over my life.
God your word says, by your stripes I am healed!
I speak life and good health over my life!
Lord not my will but your will be done!

Mathew 7:7-8 (NKJV)

"Ask, and it will be given to you; seek, and you will find; knock, and it will be opened to you. 8 For everyone who asks receives, and he who seeks finds, and to him who knocks it will be opened."

What would you like for God to do for you? Tell God what you want as it pertains to your life and your health?

_____

_____

_____

_____

_____

_____

_____

_____

_____

_____

_____

_____

_____

_____

_____

_____

_____

_____

_____

_____

_____

_____

Matthew 17:20 New King James Version (NKJV)

So Jesus said to them, "Because of your unbelief; for assuredly, I say to you, if you have faith as a mustard seed, you will say to this mountain, 'Move from here to there,' and it will move; and nothing will be impossible for you.

You must have faith that God will move on your behalf write here what you are believing God will do in your life!

_____

_____

_____

_____

_____

_____

_____

_____

_____

_____

_____

_____

_____

_____

_____

_____

_____

_____

_____

_____

_____

_____

_____

Write your own prayer/s to God about your individual situation and as I write this book if it be His will I touch and agree with you!

_____

_____

_____

_____

_____

_____

_____

_____

_____

_____

_____

_____

_____

_____

_____

_____

_____

_____

_____

_____

_____

_____

_____

_____

_____

How do you feel after you have prayed?

_____
_____
_____
_____
_____
_____
_____
_____
_____
_____
_____
_____
_____
_____
_____
_____
_____
_____
_____
_____
_____
_____
_____
_____
_____
_____

Your Death Sentence Is Not Your Demise!

Father God in the name of Jesus I come to you asking that you touch the person that is reading this book with your finger of love. I pray God that you heal them from every manner of sickness and diseases. I speak healing and wholeness in Jesus! Satan I rebuke you and command you to take your hand off of the person reading this book. God search out every need and fulfill it. Cover them with your blood Jesus so they may be able to stand. God give them the strength to fight for their life as I am doing. Everyday God give them hope and added faith. Help them to understand that the road is not easy but with you they can run this race. Bless God the ones who take care of them. Give them the strength they need to be caretakers. God we know it is not easy seeing a love one this way but give them courage to stand with them. I bind up sickness! I loose healing! I bind up depression and loose Joy! Give them the faith they need God to stand flat foot and say, I SHALL LIVE AND NOT DIE! AMEN! So fight! **FIGHT FOR YOUR LIFE!**

The Bible say's in Romans 10:9 (NKJV)

"that if you confess with your mouth the Lord Jesus
and believe in your heart that God has raised Him from the dead,
you will be saved".

That's all you have to do to come into the knowledge of God!
Make a decision to give God all of your hurt, pain, sickness, worry
and doubt and replace it with Peace, Love, Joy, Long suffering,
and most of all Faith!
YOU SHALL LIVE AND NOT DIE BUT DECLARE THE
WONDROUS WORKS OF THE LORD IN YOUR LIFE!
BELIEVE IT AND DECREE IT OVER YOUR LIFE!
LIFE AND DEATH IS IN THE POWER
OF YOUR OWN TONGUE!
SPEAK IT OVER YOUR LIFE STARTING TODAY!

REFERENCES

Elisha, H. A. (n.d.). Down at the Cross Glory to His Name. [print]. Retrieved from http://www.hymntime.com/tch/htm/d/o/w/downattc.htm

Glory to His Name Elisha A. Hoffman, pub.1878 copyright status is Public Domain.

Issac Watts, R. E. (n.d.). Alas, and did my Savior bleed. [print]. Retrieved from https://www.hymnal.net/en/hymn/h/999 This hymn was found in the Public Domain, thank you to Hymnary.org as the source.

The Holy Bible New King James Version. (1994). Nashville, Tennessee, United States of America: Thomas Nelson. Retrieved February 1, 2017

ABOUT THE AUTHOR

Valawaugn Blackmon McCain is by the grace of God a twenty-one year Astrocytoma Brain Tumor Cancer survivor and a mother of three. She has lived and faced some unbelievable challenges and now has come to share her story with you. She has an urgency in her heart to tell people diagnosed with incurable diseases to FIGHT FOR THEIR LIFE! She wants to inspire you with her story, so that you will see that even though there may be gray skies now the sun will shine again if you only believe and Never Give Up!

www.ingramcontent.com/pod-product-compliance
Lightning Source LLC
Chambersburg PA
CBHW020410290526
45785CB00005B/2491